DEDICATION

I dedicate this book to my kids. You three will always be my inspiration and my source of strength. I know with you, anything is possible.

Table of Contents

DIY Fat Burning Guide: Lose Weight Now and Easily

An Easy and Effective Guide to Shed off Those Unwanted Fats

By: Alice Campbell

9781634289726

PUBLISHERS NOTES

Disclaimer – Speedy Publishing LLC

This publication is intended to provide helpful and informative material. It is not intended to diagnose, treat, cure, or prevent any health problem or condition, nor is intended to replace the advice of a physician. No action should be taken solely on the contents of this book. Always consult your physician or qualified health-care professional on any matters regarding your health and before adopting any suggestions in this book or drawing inferences from it.

The author and publisher specifically disclaim all responsibility for any liability, loss or risk, personal or otherwise, which is incurred as a consequence, directly or indirectly, from the use or application of any contents of this book.

Any and all product names referenced within this book are the trademarks of their respective owners. None of these owners have sponsored, authorized, endorsed, or approved this book.

Always read all information provided by the manufacturers' product labels before using their products. The author and publisher are not responsible for claims made by manufacturers.

This book was originally printed before 2014. This is an adapted reprint by Speedy Publishing LLC with newly updated content designed to help readers with much more accurate and timely information and data.

Speedy Publishing LLC

40 E Main Street, Newark, Delaware, 19711

Contact Us: 1-888-248-4521

Website: http://www.speedypublishing.co

REPRINTED Paperback Edition: ISBN: 9781634289726

Manufactured in the United States of America

CHAPTER 1- INTRODUCTION

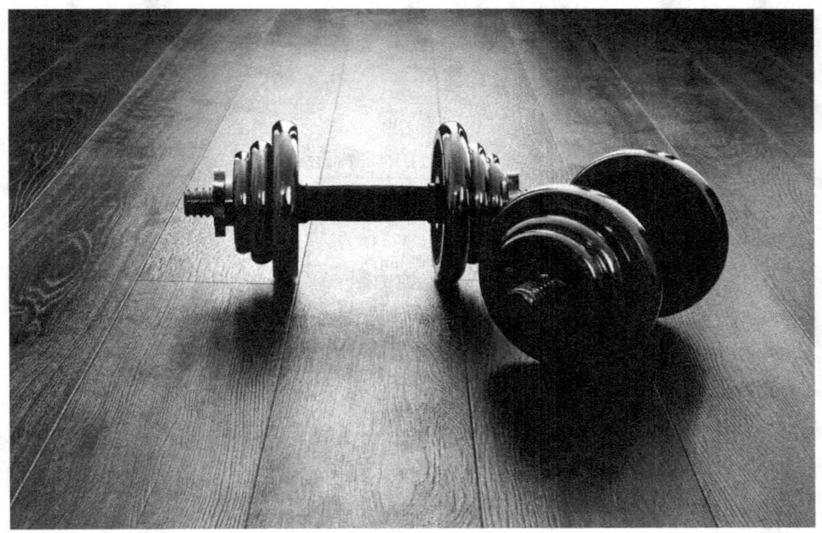

With the alarming rates of diseases that affect people nowadays, it is important for people to consider improving their physical fitness.

Unfortunately, with the wide variety of foods that surround the market at present, it can be challenging for some to avoid or neglect their cravings on their favorite foods.

However, what they don't know is that not all foods are healthy for improving one's fitness. Some of them can cause health risks, which are not a good thing most particularly if you aim to be physically fit. That is why it is wise for everyone to choose healthy foods wisely.

If you have decided to take up exercising to improve your fitness, well, congratulations! It is because empowering your fitness is the most vital step that will lead you to the "new" you! Now, the only thing that you should do is to stick with your plan and learn the basics of fitness.

There are various reasons why some people decide to incorporate physical fitness in their lives. Whether you are aiming to lose your weight, gain size or enhance you well-being, empowering your fitness can be the key for a healthier living.

The basics of fitness revolve around improving your nutrition and doing exercises. In order for you to achieve success in improving your fitness, you need to exert 100% effort and commitment. When you think of fitness, it is vital for you to take a peek at the big picture.

You have to take note that fitness is not just about endurance, strength or fat content, but also it's the combination of those factors. You can be strong, but you have no endurance. You may have endurance, but you might be less flexible.

In fitness, you need to aim for balance. There are five components that make a good fitness. Proficiency in these components will give you long- term benefits and value to your overall well-being and fitness. These components are as follows:

• Aerobic Endurance- repetitive or rhythmic activities placed an increase oxygen demand on your body systems, lungs, and heart. Big muscle groups can be used in various activities including cycling, jogging or walking. The aim of this component is to train other muscles and heart to use oxygen efficiently, which permits exercise to continue for a long period of time.

• Muscular Strength- It is the capacity of the muscles of your body to produce a huge amount of force to utilize anaerobic energy. This energy produces a short term burst of energy and will not require oxygen. Anaerobic energy comes after the carbohydrates were burned, which is needed in replenishing the system.

• Muscular Endurance- It is the measure of how your muscles can repetitively generate force to maintain the activity. This is use of the raw strengths. When compared other components, this combines both anaerobic and aerobic energy.

• Flexibility- This is ability of a person to stretch. You can increase your flexibility through stretching elastic fibers beyond their limits and maintaining the stretched muscles for several moments. Your fibers will adjust to the new limits. With an improved flexibility, the risk of experiencing injury will decrease while you are exercising and increasing your performance. Yoga and swimming are some of the exercises that require greater flexibility.

• Body Composition- This will show you the percentage of bone, muscles, and fats in your body. These percentages will give you a

view on your fitness and health in relation your body's health, age, and weight. Fat and weight are used together most of the time, but the truth is, they're not interchangeable. If you are overweight, it doesn't imply obesity. In fact, there are lots of physically fit people who are overweight because of gaining muscles. But, if you are over fat, you pose health risks that may range to high blood pressure, diabetes, and heart disease.

CHAPTER 2- FITNESS AND YOUR WELL-BEING

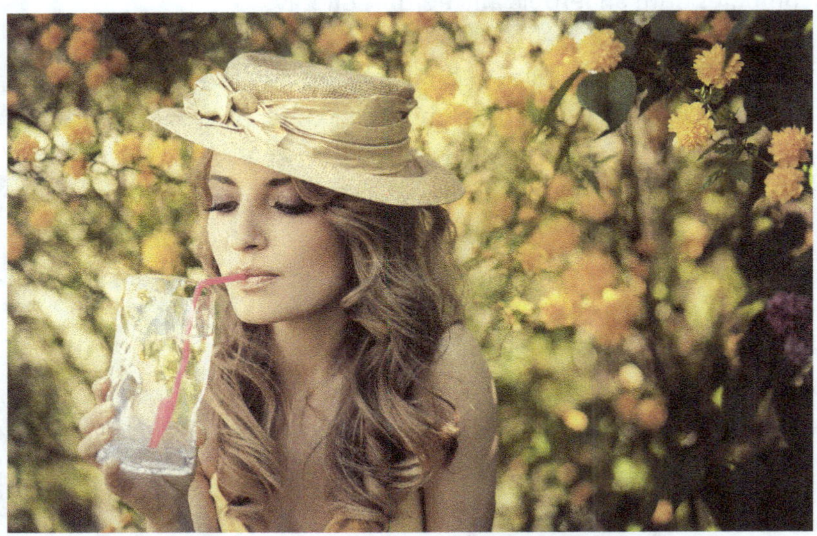

Based from the statements of experts, fitness reflects on one's muscular strength, body composition, and cardio-respiratory endurance.

Some contributors of one's physical wellbeing may include bodyweight management, avoiding unhealthy foods, and proper nutrition. Unfortunately, there is an alarming rate of increasing health risks, which also cause the overall fitness of a person to fail.

There are various factors that reduce the fitness of a person. These factors are as follows:

Influence

Fitness is said to be influenced by your own actions. Every person has the power to change the level of his or her overall fitness condition through the implementation of changes and by living a healthy and happy lifestyle. Many people will differ when it comes to their fitness level as it depends on the genetics and commitment of each person. Physical activities can help you in various ways and one of these ways is that this can help you avoid certain diseases, obesity, and other health conditions.

Change Your Routine

When working out, it is always essential to make some changes in your routine. One's body needs to keep guessing. This is because if your body is used to your daily routine, this will just result to some issues that may affect your fitness. Take note, altering your daily routine can be the key to your success. For example, if you are doing weight lifting repetitively, it will become much easier for your body to do it. However, if you will add a little twist on your daily exercises, you will surely empower your fitness.

If you are doing exercises for enhancing your cardio, don't just stick on one kind of cardio exercises. Alternate them every week and try other exercises that can contribute on your cardio workout. With this strategy, you won't just be able to increase your fitness, but also your cardio will also boost.

Nutrition

Some people don't realize that eating healthy foods can make a huge difference in increasing the level of your fitness. Whether you aspire to be a runner or you just want to lose weight, picking the right and healthy foods will assist you when making changes on your health. If you are aiming to lose weight, the best way to achieve your goals is by controlling your eating habits. Adding vegetables, grains, and more fruits is best for you. Considering smaller meals will also provide you results in the long run.

If you are having training for racing, the right way to fuel up your body is imperative. You have to get the best amount of carbohydrates and protein for maximum results. Fueling up your body with these minerals will give you more stamina for your race day.

Water

According to a particular health organization, one's body weight is made of sixty percent water. Since the body of a person depends on water, you need to drink enough amount of water to maintain the level of your body fluid even if you have done various activities. Drinking enough amount of water can also help you avoid dehydration, which may cause you to feel tired as you don't have much energy to consume. Water can help you eliminate toxins in your body and transports nutrients to each of your body cells.

Stress

Stress has a lot of effects in one's body. It may cause pains and aches that come from the tense muscles. Stress can also affect your skin. Men may suffer from various sexual problems while women may experience painful menstrual cycle. Heart disease and high blood pressure may also stem from stress. If you are experiencing too much stress, you might not achieve all your goals in fitness.

Alcohol and Drugs

The use of different recreational drugs can cause damage to one's brain cells. You have to take note that the body of each person loses its resistance to several diseases and may cause coordination issues. Alcohol, on the other hand, can cause damage to one's heart, liver, and pancreas. This can also cause increase in health risks and high blood pressure. Both can also affect the mood, memory, and body coordination.

What is True Fitness?

Fitness means different things. It may mean being able to do various physical activities or it may mean having the right amount of strength and energy. It may also be related to health. Once you get fit, your health will improve.

You don't need to become an athlete for you to get fit. Athletes are required to reach a high level of fitness, and ordinary people only need to walk for a few hours or do several exercises to reach the right fitness level.

Even if you have a busy schedule, you can have the chance to be physically fit. The only thing that you need to know is what fitness is all about and how you can become one of the physically fit individuals.

Fitness was defined as the set of attributes, which people achieve or have to do the different physical activities. But, you have to take note that whatever physical activity you're involved with, this does not define the level of your fitness. There are various components of fitness that you must be aware. These components will help you measure your fitness level.

Assessing your fitness level is important. These following components of fitness can be a huge help:

Cardio-Respiratory Endurance

Cardio-respiratory endurance is one's power of his or her respiratory and circulatory systems to generate sufficient energy that will fuel you up in order for you to do all your physical activities. In order for you to boost cardio-respiratory endurance, you need to keep your heart into the safe level that will sustain you when you are walking, running, swimming, bicycling, etc.

The activity you prefer doesn't need to be difficult when you are improving cardio-respiratory endurance. If possible, start slowly, and gradually perform on the much intense phase.

Muscular Strength

Muscular strength is one's ability of his or her muscles to exert force during physical activities. The key to make your muscles much stronger is by doing some activities that will let you boost your resistance. If you want to gain muscles and increase your muscle strength, try exercising lifting weights or take stairs rapidly.

Muscular Endurance

This is the ability of the body muscles to continue performing without fatigue. To enhance your muscle endurance, try dancing, walking, bicycling or jogging.

Body Composition

Body composition refers to fat, bone, muscle, and some parts of the body. The total body weight of a person may not change easily time. But, bathroom scales don't assess how much of your body weight contain fats and lean mass. That is the reason why it is essential for you to consider managing your weight.

Flexibility

Flexibility is said to be the motion's range around joints. If you are flexible, you can help you avoid injuries. If you want to boost up flexibility, you must try activities that will test your muscles. Basic stretching programs and swimming can be the best options that you can consider.

CHAPTER 3- FITNESS IS EASY – PERCEPTION OF THE MIND

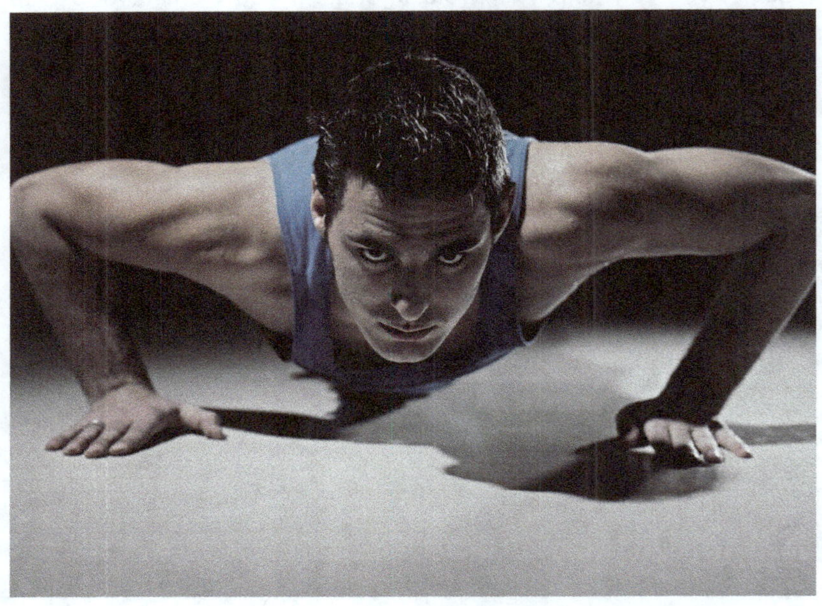

For the past few years, the industry of fitness has changed rapidly. High-tech gyms were established and almost everything was changed. However, even if there are lots of things in fitness industry that have gone drastic changes, you must bear in mind that the key to meet all your fitness goals still remain in your mind. Because of this, you need empowered fitness mindset. But, what is empowered fitness mindset all about?

Empowered fitness mindset revolves around having the right mindset to achieve what you want to increase the level of your fitness. At present, it is easy to say that you can do all your goals. But, once you have started to take action, it is never difficult for you to quit than to stay on track. Some people want to be healthy and fit. But, the problem is, they want to do it overnight, which is impossible to achieve as it requires time and effort. There is no quick solution to empower fitness. You must start first by having the right mindset.

There are several factors that affect one's mindset and these are some of them:

The Mindset

• Motivation- If you lack strong motivation, the tendency is that you might not be able to reach the things that you want to achieve. If the level of your motivation was high at the very first stage, you must maintain it once you have started your hard work. The reason behind it is that when your motivation level reduced, this will just fail you and you won't get what you want for empowering your fitness. So, seek for the best way to reaffirm your motivation.

• Remove Fear- Having fear of not being able to achieve may reduce your confidence. Accepting negativity in yourself may not be a great help as this may just lead you to the wrong path, which is failure. Therefore, if you want to get all your fitness goals, you must stop comparing yourself to other people because you can do better than them.

• It is More Than a Cardio- When working out to improve your fitness, overcoming some problems that you will encounter is never been easy. But, this does not mean that you have to give up. Rather than quitting, find ways that will work for you. Try to create some improvements by adapting changes on your lifestyle. Track things including water consumption, nutrition, time spent, body measurements, and sleep times.

These things may not be important to you, but they have a huge role in improving the level of your fitness. This will also give you the best mindset in reaching your fitness goals. With this, your confidence will also increase.

• Seek for a Training Partner or Group- There are some people who want to have someone that they can count on whenever they are working out. It is because this motivates them. If you are one of those types of persons, then it is wise to seek for a training partner or a group of fitness enthusiasts. This will help you avoid negativity and you will always enjoy working out as the atmosphere is good.

• Track and Monitor Progress- Tracking and monitoring progress in all fields of fitness and health will always let you stay on the top of the game. It will also boost your confidence and determination. So, keeping a journal of your daily progress can be helpful.

Giving up is easy especially if you haven't seen any results of your hard work. If you are facing some obstacles when improving your fitness, you must seek for the best way to face such obstacles bravely as this is what empowered fitness mindset all about.

Fitness Ideas

With the advancement of today's technology, there is no wonder that it has also changed the fitness industry. Its impact has brought good and bad things to fitness and the way people aim to increase their level of fitness. However, even if there are new fitness ideas available at present, some still think that traditional fitness ideas are much better. So, what is better between traditional fitness ideas and new age ideas?

What's New

Both traditional fitness ideas and new age ideas have pros and cons. Depending on the preference of a person, he or she can choose between the available ideas in today's market. Whatever you choose between traditional fitness ideas and new age ideas, the results will still depend on how you worked hard in empowering your fitness.

Traditional fitness ideas rely on using the available gym equipment and having proper nutrition. New age ideas, on the contrary, revolve on using the new concepts of numerous fitness experts by incorporating various approaches, programs, methods, and so on. Both can offer you benefits and may help you increase your fitness level.

New age has brought drastic changes to the fitness industry. Currently, in order for people to get fit, there are available supplements that can be used during workout or while you are under a particular program.

These supplements can be organic and artificial. These types of supplements are proven and effective. However, if you want to be successful with what you want to achieve, you must consider the one that will not fail you and will bring positive effects on your body.

Organic supplements are said to be the best one that you can consider especially if you want to empower your fitness holistically.

When compared to the traditional fitness ideas, new age ideas have opened doors of a wide collection of options. With the available concepts on how to improve one's fitness, you can incorporate a combination of the available ideas in the market today.

You can always any ideas when empowering your fitness. As long as it will keep you on the right track and will give you results in the long run, there is no need to worry about what you have chosen.

Even if there are new ideas for fitness nowadays, traditional fitness ideas still play a huge role in empowering one's fitness as they serve as the foundation of the new age fitness ideas. Without the traditional fitness ideas, new age fitness ideas will not exist.

How to Set Goals

People are always told to think big. Go for gold and reach for the stars. But, when it comes to fitness, you must learn a much calculated approach in order for you to attain your goals effectively. Empowerment for fitness means setting goals that are attainable and much realistic. So, how can you set your fitness goals?

The road to success in empowered fitness is not impossible to reach. The only way you can achieve success is by starting to set your goals. If you don't know how to set goals, here are some of the best ways to do it:

True Fitness For You

• Take Your Time- When setting goals for empowering your fitness, you don't need to rush. You can always take your time because you rule on your rules. You just need to focus for you to determine the goals that you want for your fitness.

• Make Your Goals Specific- Some people think that resolutions and goals are interchangeable. But, the truth is, resolutions imply that you're deciding something while goals are specific actions, which you want to take. For instance, the phrases "get healthy" is not specific. There are several ways for you to get healthy. This may include stopping smoking, eating the right foods, getting exercises, and so on. If you want a specific goal, you have to define exactly what you really want to do to empower your fitness.

• Make Your Goals Measurable- When you are setting goals, you must know how to keep track of your progress. Making this concrete won't only help you to stay on track, but also, this can give you motivation while reaching every step on your milestones.

• Make Sure That Your Goals are Attainable- This does not mean that you need to set your bars high just to shoot for the stars. However, there are cases that people set goals that are difficult to attain, which will just lead them to discouragement and failure. This is the reason why there are many people who are giving up when reaching their goals. So, when setting goals, see to it that they are attainable in order for you to avoid anything that will just trigger you to give up.

• Make Your Goals Much Realistic- If you are not a runner, running a marathon is an example of unrealistic goal. This does not mean that you can't do one. But, if you want to see to it that your goals are something that you will achieve, you need to asses yourself today to make it more realistic.

• Set a Time Frame- Setting a time frame can also be helpful. Without setting a deadline, you won't be motivated in doing your physical activity.

Setting goals wisely can make a difference. But, this may not mean that you will not experience failure. You still need to strive in order for you to achieve success.

CHAPTER 4- EMPOWER YOUR MIND FOR FITNESS

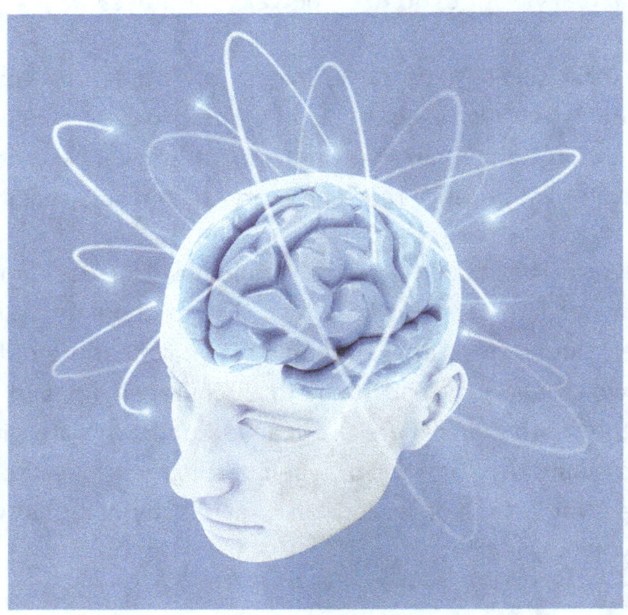

The beginnings are always tough, but if you have the right empowerment mindset for fitness, there is no way that you won't achieve all your fitness goals in your set time frame.

That is the reason why you need to consider creating a mindset that will serve as your motivation for achieving your goals. So, why do you need to adopt the right mindset for fitness?

There are many reasons why a proper mindset is important in empowering your fitness. Many people choose to give up when improving their fitness level because they think it is the best way to get rid of the obstacles they are facing. Well, it is true at some point.

But, what they don't know is that giving up will reduce their confidence to try again and reach for the stars.

Being Empowered

It is easy to start achieving your fitness goals, but it is hard to stay on the road most particularly if there are challenging obstacles that you need to face once you have started to do some workout. However, with an empowered mindset for fitness, you can do beyond limits. The reason behind it is that you will be motivated no matter how hard the challenge is.

Another reason why you must adopt empowerment mindset for fitness is that there are cases that some seek for quick fixes for increasing their fitness level. It is not an issue to seek for an easy approach. But, in order for you to achieve success, you must learn in a hard way for you to understand the real meaning of empowerment for fitness.

There are various things that you can consider when adopting empowerment mindset for fitness. First, you need to make sure that you have set goals with the use of your own approach. You may also take for consideration on the different approaches that you can use for setting proper fitness mindset.

However, when creating your own mindset, you need to take note of your needs or preferences. Take note, each person has his or her own wants or needs especially when it comes to leveling up their fitness. If you don't want to fail, you must start by making the right mindset.

Second, you must take actions on your goals. You will never achieve success if you will not start taking actions on your goals. This will serve as the key to the road of success. So, learn the best time to take actions as they may matter in the long run.

There are some reasons why you must adopt empowerment on your mindset for fitness. With this, you will not get healthy. But also, you will have the power to have a defense for diseases or illnesses that may reduce your fitness. So, why wait for a perfect time? Know and understand the reasons behind adopting empowerment mindset for fitness.

Tips for Becoming Empowered for Fitness

One of the most essential things that you can do for your fitness is by engaging in various physical activities. Exercising regularly can lower health risks and may improve your overall health and fitness condition. That is the reason why empowering fitness is vital not just for athletes, but also for those who want to avoid illnesses.

There are many ways to become empowered for fitness. If you want to be fit, you can consider the following:

Aerobic Exercise

Exercises including swimming, walking, bicycling, and jogging can help you strengthen your heart as this will keep you pumping for a long period of time. Aerobic exercise can also assist you in managing your blood pressure and energy levels.

Strength Training

Resistance or strength training can help you build stamina, which will allow you to replace body fats with lean muscle mass that encourage one's body to burn more calories efficiently. This training can also help you counteract those muscles you have lost while doing exercises like pull-ups and pushups.

Fruits and Veggies

A healthy balanced diet, which includes lots of vegetables and fruits can help you promote high levels of physical fitness because they provide the most essential nutrients and minerals to one's body. However, you have to take note that not all vegetables and fruits are healthy and nutritious. That is why you need to pick wisely to get results.

Stretching

In a fitness program, one of the most vital elements is stretching. Stretching can help your body improve your circulation. Stretching can also relieve stress and provides better posture.

Outlook

Healthy diet and regular exercise can help you to empower your fitness. If you consider your personal goals, you will surely get results in the long run. But, before you start your fitness program, you must first consult an expert to know your overall health condition.

The Good And Bad About The Empowerment Mindset For Fitness

Although being physically fit is having a good overall health condition, there are also some advantages and disadvantages that you need to know about empowering fitness. But, even if fitness has its own drawbacks, its benefits still outweigh the bad things about it. For that reason, empowerment mindset for fitness is important.

The Good And Bad

The benefits of fitness are many especially if you have incorporated empowerment mindset to reach your goals. These include greater strength, improved appearance, increased energy, better health, more positive mood and attitude, and better health. Some of the benefits of fitness include the following:

1. Reduces Health Risks- People who are physically fit can fight against the attack of various diseases or illnesses including the chronic diseases.

2. Provide Better Health- Having a high level of fitness can increase both the strength and size of your heart. This will allow your heart to pump more blood, which become more efficient. This will also lower blood pressure and lower pulse, which may increase your lifespan.

3. Lower the Level of Your Cholesterol- One of the benefits of empowered fitness is that this can help you control the level of your cholesterol. It can help you reduce the amount of bad cholesterol in your body and maximize the number of good cholesterol.

4. Build Stronger Ligaments, Joints, and Bones- If you are physically fit, your muscles will be strengthened. It can also lower the risk of bone diseases. There are also studies that show that being physically fit can help you reduce osteoporosis' severity.

5. Improve the Quality of Your Sleep- One of the main benefits of fitness is that it can help you sleep better. Studies show that those who are regularly exercising can fell asleep easily and they sleep longer compared to those who don't get enough exercise.

There are other benefits of fitness that you will get once you start to take the road of empowered fitness. Overall, fitness can improve the quality of your life and will let you live in a much healthier life.

Bad Things about Empowerment Mindset for Fitness

Although there are many reasons why people consider leveling up their fitness, there are also some problems that may popped up when you start to empower fitness. However, this may depend on the overall health condition of a person.

One of the bad things about empowerment mindset for fitness is that others might not consider following their set deadline when reaching their goals. But, if you have motivation, you can easily avoid it. Another bad thing about it is that some people might choose to give up instead of pursuing their goals. Nevertheless, even if empowerment mindset for fitness may bring negative things for people, its offered benefits are still unbeatable.

CHAPTER 5- DIY FITNESS – AEROBICS

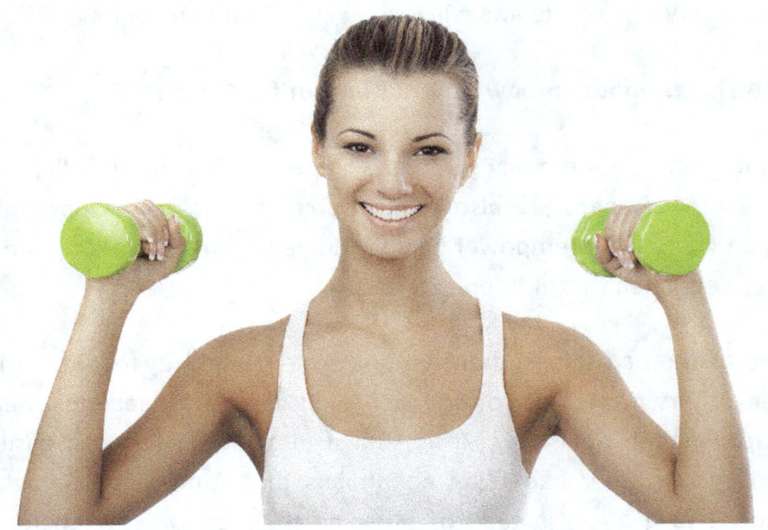

Benefits Of Aerobic Exercise

We are always reminded that exercise could do wonders for the body. Aerobics, a kind of exercise which helps your body use more oxygen while maintaining your target heart range, can definitely help a person live longer and healthier. There are studies showing that 30 minutes of aerobics every day would benefit the body a lot.

Performing regular aerobic exercises would gradually make the heart larger. A bigger and larger heart would be able to provide more oxygenated blood which can be used by the muscles. This could also mean more energy whether for longer or shorter periods of exercise or physical activities.

• Weight loss

Aerobics and any kind of physical activity could surely help control and reduce weight. It is most successful when combined with a healthy diet. Including physical activity and exercise with your daily routine will surely help you achieve better built, healthy lifestyle and increase in energy.

Aerobics would help your body burn the calories consumed and prevent them from becoming accumulated fats.

• Stronger resistance against sickness

Aerobics can boost the body's immune system. This would prevent illnesses like colds and flu from happening. It could also help the body manage existing health problems like high blood pressure and blood sugar. Excessive weight and obesity could cause serious health problems like diabetes, heart disease and stroke. Aerobics could help in reducing the risks of these diseases. This kind of exercise could help in clearing the arteries of the heart from bad cholesterol.

• Elderly benefits

Aging could have different effects on the body and exercise could help you deal with these changes. It could help your body become stronger and more mobile when you grow old.

Common problems of the elderly would be flexibility and mobility. Aerobics and maintaining other forms of exercise even when older would help reduce these problems.

• Increase in stamina and energy

Contrary to what some people think, aerobics and exercise wouldn't leave you breathless and less energetic. It could boost your stamina and energy. Continuous and regular exercise could result to muscle development and increase in body endurance. Aside from that, aerobics could also reduce fatigue and decrease shortness of breath. Aerobics could help the body achieve better sleep at night, making the person more energetic and fresh the next day.

• Promote better mental health

Exercise does not only calm and help the body, it could also help in boosting a mood of a person. Achieving better health and physical results through aerobics could increase self- esteem and self-confidence. It is even used to reduce stress, anxiety and depression.

Aerobics have numerous benefits. In fact, some would say that aside from physical and mental benefits, aerobics could also help in improving sexual performance. There are also different types of aerobic exercises which could capture the interest of people with different ages and characteristics.

However, aerobics may not be safe for everybody. Those with certain illnesses and those that are pregnant should take necessary precautions when performing aerobic exercises. Before trying any aerobic routine, it is important to consult with a doctor first especially if you have an existing or past medical condition.

Different Types Of Aerobic Exercises

Aerobics is one of the most popular types of exercises in the market. Its use of music, dance, equipment and other facilities have contributed to its popularity. Aerobic exercises are workouts that intend to increase the heart rate for a period of time. This would cause the body to have higher intake of oxygen which would result into better blood circulation, weight loss, faster calorie and fat burning.

Other physical activities can also be considered as aerobic workouts, like swimming, running, walking, jogging, and cycling. An aerobic exercise would start with a 5 to 10 minutes of warm- up stretching and exercises. After the warming-up, the routine proper would follow, lasting for about 20 to 30 minutes. The last part of the workout will be the cooling-down process.

There are different types of aerobic exercises for different levels of individuals. Skill, health and comfort are things to be considered when choosing what type of aerobic exercise would fit with the individual's needs and abilities. Some of the types are :

• Low-impact aerobics

As the name implies, low-impact exercises don't include activities which could harm the bones and joints like jumping and bouncing. Exercises performed had lower intensity, thus reducing the risks of injuries and leg overuse. In this exercise, one or both feet should always be in contact with the ground.

With low-impact routine, you do not start with a high note. An individual could start performing the exercises on a slower rate and gradually increase its intensity. Low-impact aerobics is ideal for seniors, obese and overweight individuals and of course, pregnant women.

• High impact aerobics

High impact aerobic exercises use different movements. It could include jumping, turning, shuffling, doubling, etc. This kind of workout intends to develop the abdominal area, calf, and also the cardiovascular system. If an individual is agile and active prior to working out, then high-impact aerobics may be the best option. But for beginners, slower and low-impact exercises is recommended first. When the individual is already comfortable with this low-impact level, then it would be safe to proceed with the second level. Keep in mind that doctor's discretion is always important.

• Step Aerobics

Step aerobics uses step benches for working out. This kind of aerobics is actually low in impact. There are studies showing that step aerobics can help a person reduce weight, given the fact that its impact is only half of the impact used when riding a bike at home. Overall, this process or workout is dedicated for the development of the lower body.

• Aerobic kickboxing

It is also called cardio boxing. This is one of the most effective workouts for losing weight. Although, aerobic kickboxing is tiring, its effects on the body are great. It could definitely help in building more energy and longer stamina. It is also called cardio boxing and can burn about 800 calories in an hour.

• Water aerobics

Another low-impact exercise but delivers huge results, whether it is for weight loss or improving over-all health. Water aerobics, according to experts, burns calories faster compared with land-exercises because of the water's resistance.

Wading In Water Aerobics

Physical activities like walking, running, dancing and swimming can be considered aerobics. Aerobics are exercises which increase the heart rate and at the same time pump more oxygen into the blood vessels. There are different kinds of aerobic exercises which can be defined based on the equipment used in the workout program. Water aerobic workout is an example of an aerobic workout.

Water aerobics or aqua aerobics can also be referred to as waterobics. This kind of workout is usually performed in a swimming pool with waist-deep water. It could be in an indoor or outdoor pool, with water temperature of 82º F to 86º F. Come to think of it, the most common form of waterobics is swimming. Water aerobics would focus on building body strength, flexibility, balance and providing a cardiovascular workout. It's one session usually lasts for about 40 to 50 minutes.

Just like any other aerobic workout, there is a five-minute warm-up and would end with five- minute cool-down. There could be floatation devices provided to the participants if the water is deep. Kickboards and water barbells are also provided to help participants afloat or can be used for exercises. Water weights and floating belts are also used to increase water resistance. Music are used during workout sessions.

When kicking off with waterobics, the most basic thing that you need is your swimsuit. There are some participants who would also use a swimming cap to keep the hair out of the face and

 special aqua shoes. These special shoes can support you ankles and also prevent your feet from slipping. They would also serve as protection against cuts and scrapes.

There are numerous benefits from including water aerobics in your lifestyle.

• Since water provides buoyancy and support to the body, there are less risks of bone and joint injury, which makes it ideal for seniors who are suffering from arthritis or back pains. Working out in water makes an individual less achy and sore after the workout. Body joints did not have any problem with maximizing its movement.

• Some would say that they experienced faster shaping and toning of muscles when doing water exercises, compared with conducting them on land. Water aerobics could help the muscles develop 12 to 14 times faster than it does when doing in land. Since water has higher density than air, it has higher resistance which is among the reasons for better muscular development and endurance

• The heart works better when doing water aerobics. Compared to activities like running or swimming, the heart rate is maintained at a lower rate.

• This is great for burning calories and losing weight. Walking for instance, when done on land can burn about 135 calories in half an hour. If performed in water, you could burn by as much as 264 calories for the 30-minute session.

• Aqua aerobics are great for those who have arthritis, osteoporosis and pregnant because the workouts are actually gentle enough for joint movements but quick enough to build muscle mass. Still, if a person has the following medical conditions, expert's advise is still important.

Even with all the benefits, water aerobics is still not perfect. Since it would require the use of facilities and equipment, water aerobics exercise tend to be more expensive. Some health insurance providers could provide coverage for the aqua aerobics as long as it is recommended by the attending physician.

Chapter 6- Different Types of Aerobic for your DIY Fitness

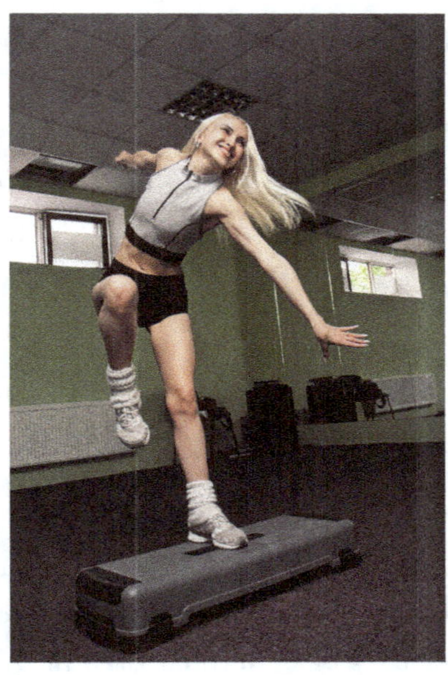

Aerobics is one of the ways to lose weight and reduce risks of sickness and complications as a result of obesity and being overweight. It will also improve overall health.

Aerobics could help in pumping more oxygen into the blood vessels, which can increase metabolism and burn more fat and calories. Aerobics literally means oxygen. Aerobic exercises are designed to increase oxygen intake. This practice would burn fat and improve health and fitness.

According to studies, about 300,000 adult deaths in the United States can be attributed to the lack of physical activity and unhealthy eating habits. About two thirds of adults in the U.S. are overweight, while about one-third of the adult population are obese.

Adults are not the only ones suffering from weight problems. Children and teens with obesity have increased for the last years because of changes in lifestyle.

Would it be possible then to lose weight just by breathing alone?

Breathing is a crucial aspect in different kinds of exercises. In fact, in yoga, breathing properly is important. Breathing exercises could even remove stress and relax the body and mind.

Breathing for weight loss is practiced by several aerobic breathing programs. Each program would have their own technique and their own advice.

However, it is important to understand that there is no weight loss program or pill that could produce dramatic results overnight. Obesity and being overweight cannot be resolved by aerobic breathing alone. Of course, proper diet and exercise is still crucial to battle the pounds away. Aerobic breathing can supplement these weight loss programs to acquire better results.

Most of us would only use about 20% of our lung capacity, while 70% of toxic elimination in our body happens when we breathe. Aerobic breathing helps our body maximize its potential. By breathing properly for about 20 minutes a day, you can bring drastic results in your health.

The guiding principle is that breathing can cleanse your body. It could help in flushing out waste, toxins and other pollutants from your body. Diaphragmatic deep breathing techniques could help in reducing cellulite, improve skin tone, blood circulation, digestion and even sleep.

With aerobic breathing, all you have to do is sit up straight, exhale from the lungs and inhale through the nose. Breathing should be able to stretch the lungs to its capacity. When exhaling, make sure to force out all the air in the lungs.

Hold breathing for a while and then pull your stomach in. You can do these breathing exercises about 10 to 20 times. Some would prefer doing them before proceeding with any exercise training.

Everyone wants to lose weight. But it does not mean that you should start starving yourself and become a slave to exercise machines. In the end, losing weight would still mean eating fruits, vegetables and healthy food, exercising regularly and staying or maintaining a positive outlook of life.

Whenever we are including ourselves in aerobics and weight loss programs, setting realistic goals for us to accomplish would make it easier for us and at the same time, take weight loss according to our own phase. Breathing may not be the magic beans we're looking for to look good, but it can definitely help us change into a new person.

Aerobic Dance

Aerobic dancing combines exercises and different forms of dances like ballet and jazz into an exercise routine. They are usually considered low-impact exercises and slower paced compared with other aerobic routines, although there are also fast-paced routines. Because of these characteristics, they are very ideal for those who need low-impact routines like the elderly, overweight and those who are pregnant.

What makes aerobic dance an interesting routine is, of course, its music. There are different types of music which can be used for different aerobic dances, there are different speed and style variations of aerobic dances. There are guidelines for aerobic music. It is usually about 120 to 124 beats per minute for step aerobics. For low-impact exercises, it is usually about 136 to 148 beats per minute. Beginners would dance or sweat it out with slower beats.

Aerobic dance could be classified into high-impact exercises, low-impact, step aerobics and water dance aerobics. High impact exercises, as its name implies, would involve intensive exercises which includes jumping actions synchronized with the music. Step aerobics uses the step bench, and the water aerobics is performed in waist-deep water.

Aside from the movements along with the music, aerobic dance is also combined with fast or aerobic breathing. This pumps more oxygen into the blood stream, rejuvenating the body.

Aerobic dances are usually done from 20 to 30 minutes, practiced for three times a week. The routine is performed just like rhythmic dances, with counts essential in setting the rhythm.

Before proceeding with the routine, getting warmed-up is important. It would usually last for 10 to 15 minutes. These stretching exercises will lower risks of injury and at the same time prepare the body for any extensive movement. After the routine proper, relaxing or cooling down movements for another 5 to 15 minutes will be performed to help the heart and the muscles relax.

Aerobic dancing has many benefits even though they were done or practiced in a fun way. This kind of aerobic workout is a great way to lose weight and at the same time, tone body muscles. It would also help the body develop strength among bones who carry most the body's weight and also toughen cardiovascular muscles.

Just like other exercises, aerobic dance can increase the circulation of the blood, reduce the levels of blood sugar and cholesterol. Because aerobic dancing would include proper breathing exercises, more oxygen is circulated in the heart, lungs and blood vessels which makes the body to function better, produce higher energy and stamina. Its physical benefits would also include boosting of the immune system, preparing the body against colds, flu, etc.

Aerobic dancing is also a great way to keep stress away. This could break the stressful and monotonous routine we have at home, school or in the work place. It can even allow you to develop or practice your creativity, since you can create your own dance steps or routine. If you cannot leave the house to go to a gym, you could do the aerobic exercises at home, learn the steps and pick your own song. How fun it is to stay healthy with aerobics by swaying your hips!

Aerobic Equipment

Aerobics is not only good for your body but also for your overall health. It is also a great way of losing weight and keeping the unwanted pounds away. Although aerobic exercises are good as it is like kickboxing, walking, jogging or similar routines, using aerobic equipments would make exercising more fun and at the same time burn calories faster.

There are different kinds of equipment which could be used for different aerobic exercises.

• Step bench

This is the most common equipment. The height of the step depends on the leg movements that would be used. Of course, the height would depend on the experience and expertise of the person using it. Usually, a beginner would start with a 4-inch step. As the person becomes more experienced, the height would increase to build more endurance and flexibility. One thing great about aerobic steps is that it is portable enough to be carried anywhere.

When buying a step bench, a bench with a non-slip surface will be a good idea since it would more safe. Just keep in mind that a higher step bench would mean a more intense workout.

• Stationary Bicycle

Unlike ordinary bicycles there are located only in one place. To measure the progress of the bike, an ergo meter is installed. There are even stationary bikes which have computers that contain the exercise data and sessions. These bikes have different features which influence the costs of the equipment. There are different kinds of stationary bikes, buying one does not mean you would have to pick the most sophisticated and expensive model. The needs of the user come first.

• Treadmill

Treadmills can be expensive. There are manual and motorized treadmills which can be bought from different fitness centers. There are different features included in a treadmill like the pulse monitor, bottle holder, and book rack. There are even sophisticated models which would allow you to use video and audio players to kill boredom while doing the exercises. When buying treadmill, the size is the most important factor. Check if it would be able to fit into your exercise or living room area.

• Hand weights

Lifting weights is another component of aerobic exercises. When seriously trying to build muscles, then start getting 3 lbs. and 5 lbs. weights. When using hand weights, users are recommended to use aerobic gloves to grip better. Water aerobics also have customized weights which can be used in aquatic exercises.

Whenever performing aerobic exercises, using the proper gear is important, the right clothes and shoes. Make sure that the clothes will allow the body to move easily, the shoes should be comfortable enough and keep the user balanced.

Aside from paying attention to wearing the proper working-out clothes, asking your doctor or health-care provider about any kind of recommendation with what kind of fitness equipment and program would be suitable for your needs is important. If buying fitness equipment is out of the option, then you could always sign-up for a membership in fitness centers, as long as they offer the equipment you would prefer to use.

Aerobic Kickboxing

There are different types and routines in aerobics. And one of them is aerobic kickboxing. Aerobic kickboxing should not be confused with kickboxing which is a self-defense technique. With aerobic kickboxing, which is also called cardio kickboxing, you could lose about 800 calories within an hour. Aside from losing weight, cardio kickboxing is also great in building lower and upper body strength.

Aerobic kickboxing starts just like any other kind of aerobic exercise, with a five to ten minutes of warm-up. After that, it would be the kicking and punching which would end up with another five minute cool-down. This aerobic exercise combines martial-arts, self-defense, boxing and music. A person who is performing this would be able to learn the basics of these parts. For example, basic boxing stance is taught. Punches like jabs and hooks, kicks like sidekicks are taught.

Kickboxing is thought to have originated from Muay Thai. But aside from the Thai boxing influences, aerobic kickboxing also uses karate skills to develop flexibility, strength and endurance in one cardiovascular exercise. Those who practice aerobic kickboxing would also testify that it was able to help them build their self-confidence, self-esteem, self-control and develop a positive attitude towards exercising and work-out.

In addition to that, it can also reduce levels of stress and increase the individual's stamina and energy. Imagine, learning self-defense and keeping your personal fitness in check in an hour or less in a day. But as great as it is, there should be considerations before practicing aerobic kickboxing.

• Your personal level of fitness.

Aerobic kickboxing is a high-impact aerobic routine. Those who are suffering from arthritis, tight hamstrings and inflexible back can have difficulties with this routine. And always consider getting your doctor's advice before proceeding with any kind of exercise program especially if you have an existing medical condition.

• Consider your level of expertise.

If it is your first time to do such workout, then you could always get a beginning class. After being familiar with it, you could start progressing into intermediate and advance levels. If working out with a CD/DVD or tape at home, then pay attention to the instructions and start and do the workout according to your own pace. There are moves like high-kicks which should be avoided by beginners. These moves would require flexibility which would be developed later on when you have already gotten used to the routine.

• Hydrate.

Always drink water before, during and after the workout.

• If the CD or the class runs for more than an hour, you are not obligated to work out for the entire period. An hour of aerobic exercise is enough.

• Wear clothes that would not restrict the flow of movements while exercising. Loose-fitting clothes could be a problem sometimes.

Cardio kickboxing could still put beginners at risk of joint injury. Especially, if they would be extending or using incorrect forms and stances like overextending kicks and locking joints.

Wearing weights and holding dumbbells are also not a good idea since they could also be detrimental to your joints. When performing aerobic kickboxing or any kind of aerobics, never give in to peer-pressure and excise beyond your limits or fatigue.

Keep in mind that speed, flexibility and your overall performance and fitness will increase along with regular practice.

Step Aerobics

Aerobics, developed by Dr. Kenneth Cooper in the early seventies, had become one of today's most performed exercises. Aerobics (literally "with oxygen") is basically a form of exercise to improve one's overall fitness in muscular strength, flexibility and cardiovascular health.

One of today's more popular forms of aerobics exercises is called step aerobics, introduced at the start of the 90s. The new form is an innovation of the old aerobics routine, this time having a step (a raised contraption, 6 to 8 inches high) where the aerobics performer will step on or off from time to time.

The stepping rates (it usually starts at 120 per minute) and the height of the steps (6 to 8 inches) are adjusted according to the exerciser's needs and experience. These simple step-up, step-down aerobics are as beneficial as those of more intense movements, but less damaging to the joints.

Basic moves

The basic step involves stepping one foot first and then the other on top of the step, and stepping down on the floor using the same sequence of foot movements. There is a general agreement among aerobic enthusiasts that the "right basic" is stepping right foot up, then the left, and then stepping down to the floor with the right then the left foot.

For variations, instructors switch different moves within the sequence, like changing the "right basic" to the "left basic" without in-between moves. Usually, this is done by way of "tapping" the foot instead of shifting weights.

Another form of step is called "tap-free" or smooth step. This is done with the feet always alternating and without the confusing "taps". The "taps" can sometimes make learning difficult for new aerobics students.

The instructor usually plans beforehand when to insert a switching move that maintains the natural rhythm of moves to simulate the natural shifting of weights on both legs like in walking.

From the right basics, the instructor might insert a "knee up" (lifting a knee and during the return, switches the move to the other foot) and continue with the left basics.

Sets

Usually, a set prepared by the instructor consists of many different moves with different durations. This is executed together by the whole class and usually timed to 32 beats per set. This is done in such a way that the whole set can be switched and repeated in the other leg, mirror-like.

 Basic level classes have simpler basic moves. Advanced classes sometimes incorporate dance elements like turns and stomps and whatever is in vogue.

Elements are strung together in two to three routines per class. One learns these routines in class, which will be performed at the end of the class. Most instructors offer several choices for every person's level of intensity or dance ability during the teaching of the routines.

Benefits

Step aerobics helps burn calories and maintain weight. The amount of calories that are burned depend on the intensity, speed and the duration of the aerobic exercises.

Step aerobics helps in endurance, prevents cardiovascular diseases, and improves gait and balance. It also provides flexibility training to enhance joints movements.

Finally, step aerobics helps maintain good mental health because the workouts are fun and enjoyable, and sessions certainly release stress. With a group session, a person's social life is enhanced as well.

Aerobics For Kids

It is important to teach kids early about health and fitness. Involving them in exercise and aerobics would not only help them understand health but also help them direct their energies into movements and practices that would be productive and at the same time, beneficial in the long run.

According to studies, about 25% of children and teens do not have any "vigorous physical activity." About 14% children and teens report no physical activity like walking or cycling, everyday. This can be one of the reasons why the number of children has doubled since the early 1970s. In 2000, 19% of children, 6 to 11 years old, and 17%, 12 to 19 years old, are considered overweight.

Those who are involved in physical activities, reduce the risks of developing health problems as they grow older. Exercising reduces the risks of obesity, diabetes, high blood pressure, stroke and heart disease. But making your child follow a 30 minute exercise video is no fun for your kid.

There are fitness centers that have children workout program, they would include biking, swimming, walking, marching, playing games to introduce low, moderate and high impact aerobics and physical activity.

Introducing children and teens to aerobics would help them become more active and at the same time, change their outlook towards the lifestyle they will be having as they grow old.

There are also fitness centers which offer exercise programs suitable for children and teens, based on their age, skill and of course, their fitness and personal condition.

There are also CDs and DVDs that mix an aerobic workout with dances and other fun ways. Teens and older children may enjoy dancing to hip-hop and modern dances. Some would also show interest in doing aerobic dances, kickboxing, yoga and Pilates. You could also help your child participate in school-organized sports and activities.

There are guidelines that should be kept in mind when involving your child in physical activity according to Centers for Disease Control and Prevention (1997) and the Council for Physical Education for Children (1998). Children should at least be physically active within 30 to 60 minutes on all or most of the days of the week. Moderate to vigorous activity a day should last for about 10 to 15 minutes. Playing games and activities like biking, walking, running, etc. should also be included in the child's activities.

To encourage physical activity, make sure to implement rules that would lead to healthier lifestyle. This would include setting time for watching television and computer games. Aside from that, make sure that your child would be eating meals not in front of the television or computer. This would promote or give time for parents to talk to children during meals.

The easiest way to teach and encourage children to exercise is to set an example. Obesity and overweight problems are not just children health concerns, alarmingly, a lot of adults also suffer from these health problems. The family exercising together helps the family build stronger and closer relationships. Aerobics would not only benefit your child, but the whole family as well.

The Best Types Of Aerobics

Since the 80s, aerobics took the world of exercise by storm. Different from high intensity workouts used by professional athletes before, aerobics is a moderate exercise that is effective in improving one's overall fitness.

After being developed by Dr. Kenneth Cooper, regular aerobics exercises and routines had been enhanced and were given innovations since its inception into the mainstream of modern life.

A big part of the appeal of aerobics on almost everybody is the fact that it is simply any moderate physical activity that can be performed continuously for a certain length of time.

This type of exercise works the body at the lower end of the target heart rate area, causing the heart and lungs to adapt and become strong.

Because of this, aerobics is known as the best cardio and weight-loss exercise routine. Most bodybuilders attest that aerobics provide a sustained calorie-burning effect not matched by any exercise.

The best aerobic exercise for burning fat and losing permanent weight will depend, of course, on the individual's fitness level. If one has low fitness levels (most often, people who are just starting out), walking or step aerobics would probably be best.

Some recommendations

For starters, the best aerobics would include walking, running, jumping rope, ski machines, treadmills, rowers, health riders and more.

If you are just starting out or have not been working out lately, the best starter program is walking. Even if the fat-burning potential in walking is low, this is a great routine for beginners.

In time, on the advice of your trainer and doctor, you can step up your routine. Perhaps, you can later jog and increase the intensity level in your fat-burning.

Running and cycling

Running or jogging, the logical next level after your walking is rated the best aerobic exercises by many experts. It has a high fat-burning capacity, and if done with consistency, will produce obvious results every practitioner can feel and see for themselves.

One should be on alert, though, on the danger for individuals to over-train. The name of the game is moderation, especially if you have some medical history of cardio-vascular problems. As always, consult your doctor first.

Cycling, either on a stationary bike or a real one, is another fun and excellent aerobics routine. Cross-country or mountain biking not only gives you the exercise benefits you want, but will also get you to see scenic places that can excite the mind.

Treadmills and weights

In treadmills, you can combine walking, jogging and perform resistance training as well. The possibility of doing high intensity exercise routines in treadmills makes them very effective aids in your fat-burning goals.

This is also true with other exercise gears in the gym like rowing machines. In rowing, the whole body routines can greatly help in burning calories.

On the advice of your trainer, you may add a light weight training session to your aerobics. This might be done at least thrice a week. Weight training with aerobics is a potent combination for burning fat as well as preserving and toning your muscles.

Moderation and consistency

In all of these, the main frame of mind of the exerciser should be consistency. Aerobics needs moderation. Anything more intense is another exercise program.

How-Can-Aerobics-Help-You-Lose-Weight

One of the most popular means of losing weight ever since is aerobic exercises because of its long term benefits when it comes to overall health. Although many people are living testaments to the wonders of weight loss by dieting and cutting down on important nutrients, not all of these offer certain and desirable results like aerobic exercises can.

If you are one of those who are contemplating over losing weight, then now is the time to stop entertaining the thoughts on weight loss programs or diets. It is now time to conduct a little research first on aerobic exercises to help you understand how aerobics help you lose weight and achieve can long term health benefits.

Aerobics basics

Aerobics refer to doing an activity such as a physical exercise for a longer period of time but with lesser force and effort on the part of the one who is doing it. Simply put, aerobics exercises are those that allow a person to do multi-tasking such as carrying out a conversation while doing the exercise or engaging in simple yet productive activities.

The most common forms of aerobic exercises might include simple walking, jogging, swimming and even cross country skiing. To those who cannot carry on these simple exercises religiously on their own, they can try attending aerobic classes nearby where there is an instructor to lead them.

Experts say that before you engage in any activity such as aerobic exercises please make sure that you have reviewed its requirements well. Avoid choosing activities that would not suit your health and lifestyle conditions.

Also, make sure that you have visited a registered or licensed physician first before trying on aerobic exercises and before using any weight loss product that you think might complement your activity such as food supplements, herbs, or over-the-counter medications.

What can be done?

To ensure that aerobic exercises will work for you, take time off to read and understand various issues surrounding it. You can check the Internet where there are thousands of sites that will lead you into any information you want on aerobic exercise or ask a person who you know that did this before so you can ask for first hand tips and suggestions. It will also help if you:

-record your eating habits and patterns by keeping a food journal. Updating and monitoring your food and eating patterns will help you track down the reasons behind your weight gain. Asking for professional help from a registered dietitian will make the monitoring more valid.

-indulge and give in if you are craving for a specific food or dish since being not overly- restrictive with food or favorite treats can be awarding experience. By giving into these cravings you can totally avoid eating foods that are high in calories and fats.

-engage yourself in only one daily exercise such as walking—which is the easiest form of aerobic exercise—since it is recommended by most authorities to help you lose weight while keeping your body fit and healthy. Other exercises and workouts that last 30 to 60 minutes will also help you burn unwanted fats and calories.

Aerobics During Pregnancy

Everybody can benefit from exercise, even those who are handicapped. The elderly would exhibit health improvements when performing low-impact exercises. Pregnant women would also benefit from low-impact aerobic exercises. Those who practice aerobics while pregnant would experience easier labor and child-birth.

There are also studies that showed women who have been performing aerobic exercises have reduced risk of undergoing caesarean operation/ surgery, quicker recovery whether it is physical or from postpartum depression.

These women would also shed pounds gained during pregnancy, faster. Overall, women would testify that they had healthier pregnancy compared with other women.

Exercising while pregnant does not mean that soon-to-be-mothers would carry on the same pace or exercises they were doing prior to pregnancy. Since expecting mothers are practically sustaining two lives in their bodies, they should not be exerting too much in their exercises.

Pregnant women are recommended to perform aerobic exercises for not more than 30 minutes. When exercising too much, the body temperature of both mother and child could increase.

This could cause problems with the baby, excessive heat during the first trimester could cause birth defects. While later on during second trimester, it could trigger premature birth.

To avoid hyperthermia or excessive heat, exercises can be performed early in the morning when the weather is cooler. Pregnant women should drink plenty of water and avoid exerting too much force or energy, like weightlifting.

Places like saunas and steam rooms should be avoided. As all pregnant women know, exercises which would make the abdomen and the stomach vulnerable should be avoided by all means. Jumping movements should also be avoided.

Light weight-lifting can also be practiced by pregnant women. This would be able to prepare them for carrying the baby after birth. Although, experts would always recommend that before proceeding to any kind of aerobic routine or program, doctor's advice is very important.

Other forms of exercise which could be carried out during the first trimester would include swimming, walking, and there are special aerobic programs designed for pregnant women. While exercising, it is important to keep eat and keep your body hydrated.

During the second and last trimester, the weight of the baby could have an effect on your movements. Maintaining your balance is hard since the weight could provide stress in your joints. During this time, marching in place could replace your usual exercise routine. Exercises which would require you to bend over, spin and quick turning movements can cause the mother to lose balance and result into injury.

Use caution as you move across the floor. You may want to try a prenatal water aerobics class if one is offered in your community. It offers many of the same benefits as aerobics on land- a workout for your heart and body and the camaraderie of other expectant mothers without the stress on your joints or the risk of injury or a fall.

Even though aerobics has many benefits, doctors may not recommend it to some pregnant moms especially if they show signs of preeclampsia or worsening hypertension. The American College of Obstetricians and Gynecologists (ACOG) also cautions pregnant women against aerobic exercises that would require them to lie on their backs when they're about 20 weeks pregnant. Generally, if a pregnant woman is experiencing unusual symptoms like pain, bleeding, rapid heartbeat or dizziness, exercises should be stopped.

CHAPTER 7- EQUIPMENT NEEDED FOR YOUR AEROBICS FITNESS

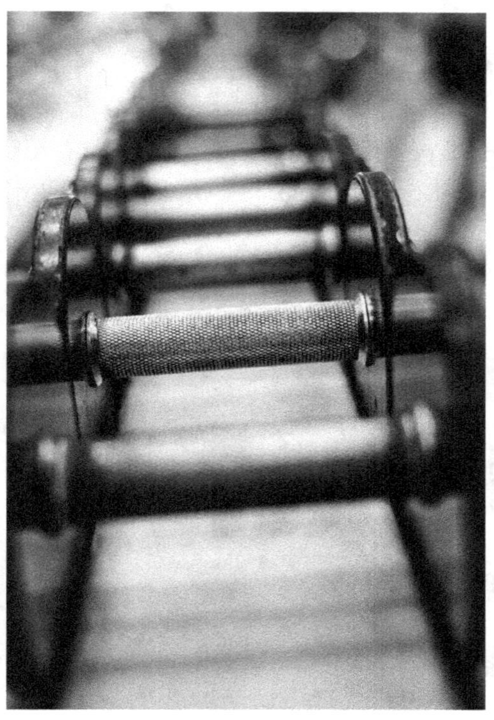

Aerobics is not only good for your body but also for your overall health. It is also a great way of losing weight and keeping the unwanted pounds away.

Although aerobic exercises are good as it is like kickboxing, walking, jogging or similar routines, using aerobic equipments would make exercising more fun and at the same time burn calories faster.

There are different kinds of equipment which could be used for different aerobic exercises.

• Step bench

This is the most common equipment. The height of the step depends on the leg movements that would be used. Of course, the height would depend on the experience and expertise of the person using it. Usually, a beginner would start with a 4-inch step. As the person becomes more experienced, the height would increase to build more endurance and flexibility. One thing great about aerobic steps is that it is portable enough to be carried anywhere.

When buying a step bench, a bench with a non-slip surface will be a good idea since it would more safe. Just keep in mind that a higher step bench would mean a more intense workout.

• Stationary Bicycle

Unlike ordinary bicycles there are located only in one place. To measure the progress of the bike, an ergo meter is installed. There are even stationary bikes which have computers that contain the exercise data and sessions. These bikes have different features which influence the costs of the equipment. There are different kinds of stationary bikes, buying one does not mean you would have to pick the most sophisticated and expensive model. The needs of the user come first.

• Treadmill

Treadmills can be expensive. There are manual and motorized treadmills which can be bought from different fitness centers. There are different features included in a treadmill like the pulse monitor, bottle holder, and book rack. There are even sophisticated models which would allow you to use video and audio players to kill boredom while doing the exercises. When buying treadmill, the size is the most important factor. Check if it would be able to fit into your exercise or living room area.

• Hand weights

Lifting weights is another component of aerobic exercises. When seriously trying to build muscles, then start getting 3 lbs. and 5 lbs. weights. When using hand weights, users are recommended to use aerobic gloves to grip better. Water aerobics also have customized weights which can be used in aquatic exercises.

Whenever performing aerobic exercises, using the proper gear is important, the right clothes and shoes. Make sure that the clothes will allow the body to move easily, the shoes should be comfortable enough and keep the user balanced.

Aside from paying attention to wearing the proper working-out clothes, asking your doctor or health-care provider about any kind of recommendation with what kind of fitness equipment and program would be suitable for your needs is important. If buying fitness equipment is out of the option, then you could always sign-up for a membership in fitness centers, as long as they offer the equipment you would prefer to use.

The Beauty Of Aerobic Exercises

Today, more and more remedies are being offered in the market for those people who would want to lose weight. Among these are weight loss remedies come in the form of products, supplements, and programs. But if there is one thing that experts would consider the safest, it would be aerobic exercises.

Before you engage in any weight loss diet, product, or program, make sure that you have full comprehension of its effects and possible side effects to avoid going back to your form after you lose weight. Being knowledgeable about these products and the possible risks associated with it can give you an idea what are the products you can take in, diets you can engage in or programs you can enroll with.

Most studies show that diets that promote weight loss of more than two pounds weekly are not safe because it increases the possibility of serious health problems compared to gradual weight loss. Medical experts also agree that losing weight at a slower rate may reduce risks of health problems that are closely associated with rapid weight loss.

Also, fad diets and quick weight loss products available today do not only ignore but totally violates the basic principles of good nutrition and various dietary guidelines. Do not be overwhelmed with the promise of quick weight loss because any claims that a person can lose weight almost effortlessly are fabricated.

These are just some of the reasons why more and more experts recommend safe means of cutting down on weight such as aerobics. Since aerobic exercises entail doing a lesser effort in an activity for a longer period of time, many say that this could be an effective tool to achieve long term health benefits.

How to keep it up

Aside serious health risks and psychological impacts brought by futile dieting, improper weight loss through the use of non-prescribed weight loss products or diets that are not proven to be effective can bring depression plus a weakened immune system.

This is why experts strongly recommend safe means of being fit and slim through aerobic exercises.

Many say that losing weight can be frustrating but a rewarding feat once you have achieved your ideal weight and figure. To help you keep up the weight that you have lost in simple aerobic exercises, here are some things that you need to debunk:

- "Low Carb Diet" is the only way for you to lose weight. This is probably one of the biggest lies being promoted by the people of weight loss industry today since by cutting out all carbo and starches will only result to lack of nutrition needed by the body especially by the muscle tissues; and

 - A lot of time is needed to work a weight loss program into your schedule. If you think that you cannot handle your weight loss all by yourself, then opt enrolling in a safe and responsible weight loss option such as aerobic classes that can fit into your schedule then you can even do other things for yourself.

The Need For Aerobics

Aerobics had been a worldwide phenomenon since the 80s, and most of the world knows about it. For the uninitiated, Dr. Kenneth Cooper (its developer) submitted the official definition to the Oxford English Dictionary.

Accordingly, aerobics is defined as "a method of physical exercise for producing beneficial changes in the respiratory and circulatory systems by activities which require meeting a modest increase of oxygen intake and so can be maintained."

Because of today's many new illnesses (hypertension, type 2 diabetes, and other cardiovascular conditions) brought about by modern man's generally inactive physical lifestyle, experts strongly recommend aerobics for everyone.

Aerobic exercise

The common definition of aerobics is simply the activity that consists of low-intensity repetitive motions of mostly the large muscles of the arms and legs for a period of time. This activity increases breathing and heart rate.

Most low-intensity activities you do during the day also fall under this category. It includes such regular activities as walking, jogging, swimming, and cycling.

For individuals who are beginners in exercise programs, or maybe have histories of health conditions, light exercise routines are recommended at first on most days of the week.

Cardiovascular benefits

Experts advise that these aerobic exercises have to be performed at moderate intensity. This level of activity is safe for almost everyone, and it still provides the desired health benefits.

Recent research brings in additional good news. It is revealed that aerobics performers can still have cardiovascular benefits even if the exercise routine (usually 30 minutes total) is broken into three or four 8-10 minute segments, as long as they are of the same intensity.

Intensity

Doctors, however, discourage infrequent bouts of high-intensity aerobics routines. It is found that this approach is not very healthy.

In the first place, reduction in risks of hypertension, high cholesterol, type 2 diabetes and other conditions depends on the total volume of the exercise done, rather than on intensity.

Higher intensity exercise activities raise your chances for muscle or joint injury. Worse, it may trigger fatal consequences because of heart rhythm disturbances.

Aerobics instructors always begin their sessions with light stretching and low-intensity movements for about 5 to 10 minutes. This warm-up routine is important to avoid injury. At the end of the routine, a similar cooling-down period for about 5 to 10 minutes is also done.

Benefits

As had been proven these years, people who engaged in regular aerobics have been known to benefit by way of lower blood cholesterol counts, lower blood pressure, toned body because of fat reduction and beneficial weight loss.

They have been known to have developed muscular and overall body endurance, have a happier disposition and moods, and a medically-certified general lower risk to cardiovascular diseases.

Common activities

The best part is the easy way on how to do your aerobics, even without going to the gym and participating in gym routines.

Doctors recommend a simple walk that totals around 10,000 steps a day. Start with something lower, and add the number of steps slowly every day until you reach your goal.

Done on a regular basis, brisk walking is guaranteed to erase your common health risks. Your need for aerobics is not be that hard to fill up.

Chapter 8- What is Adrenaline Fitness?

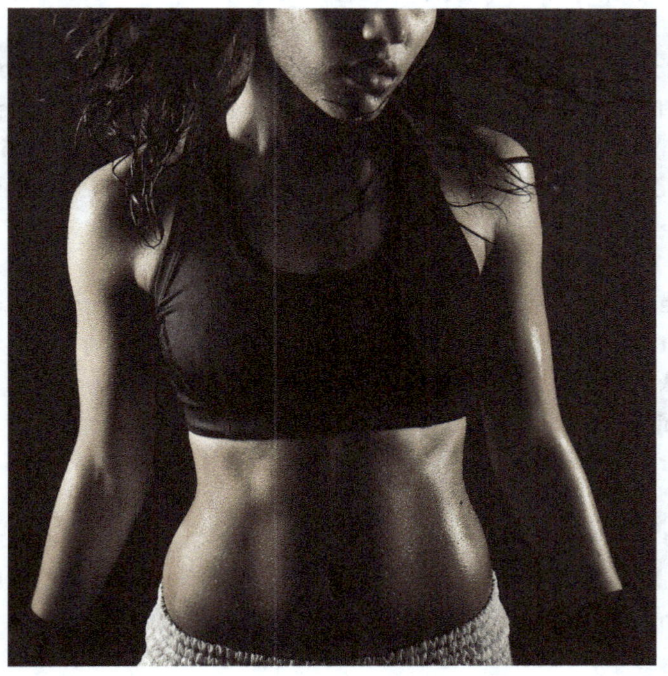

Surely, you know what adrenaline is. It's a hormone that provides you a boost in energy when you are confronted with a situation that needs vigorous physical action like when you brace yourself for a fight or flight.

The energy produced in situations such as these are often greater than normal times.

Plyometrics on other hand is known as jump training, which means that the whole fitness program is based on jumping exercises that induce your body to secrete just the right amount of adrenaline.

Another important use of adrenaline is it jumpstarts the fat burning process because, of course, energy is produced from this process.

Some of jump exercises that help increase adrenaline production are the box jump, explosive squats and double leg butt kicks.

You do not actually need a box for the box jump, stairs will do just fine. The exercise involves jumping from the lower to the next rung. You jump to the higher rung from a squatting position and immediately after landing; you get off it and repeat the movements 8 times.

The explosive squat is not difficult. You start from a regular squatting position with your feet a foot (hip width) apart. With your knees slightly bent, back straight, and butt pushed out, jump the highest you are capable of while straightening your arms upwards, repeat immediately when you land.

To do the double leg butt kicks you contract your muscles then jump high and while you are up in the air touch your butts with your heels. This is done in two sets with 8 reps.

Adrenaline, also known as "epinephrine" is a hormonal stress from adrenal glands on the kidneys. It performs a vital function in helping the body to have a reaction caused by the hostile environment.

Adrenalin rush is an abrupt increase of the adrenaline secretion from adrenal glands. It occurs if the brain connects to the glands telling that a fight-or-flight reaction is needed.

Adrenaline rush is not necessarily a physical risk but also a possible imaginary threat, failure of the heart, anxiety, brain disorder, or vigorous exercise.

Adrenaline Rush

When a person observes something exciting or intimidating, the brain communicates to the adrenal glands that adrenaline should be produced together with other hormones related to stress. Adrenal glands are responsible for creating adrenaline by transforming amino acid into dopamine.

Giving oxygen to dopamine yields noradrenalin and later on becomes adrenaline. This adrenaline joins the receptors of the arteries, heart, liver, fatty tissue, and pancreas. Afterwards, adrenaline will increase the respiration and heartbeats.

By connecting to the receptors of the liver, pancreas, fatty tissue, and muscles, it prevents the formation of insulin. It promotes the synthesis of fats and sugar by which the body uses it to kindle the fight-or-flight circumstances.

Health Effects

Adrenaline rush can produce bad effects to the health. Those people suffering from heart disease can cause their hearts to become weak. Heart muscle is made weak and there is heart attack, or heart failure to happen next.

The brain can also be affected in unhealthy manner. On-going high levels of stress will lead the brains central memory to shrink. Stress hormones promote the formation of signaling molecules responsible for the swelling of hippocampus. The stressful condition also stops the development of the new neurons.

Memory and Stress Hormones

Although adrenaline glands create a big area for the adrenaline synthesis, neurons of the brain will also form adrenaline. Very stressful situations speed up the activity of the neurons. The result can be a negative effect on the brain's memory. Stress can affect the memory storage by stimulating the main part of the brain which has the influence in storing negative feelings. Usually, people learn faster if things are played again and again in their memory. However, a single event can be enough for neurons to produce continuing networks.

Treatment

Irregular occurrences of adrenaline rush in a natural way does not need any medication. If recurring stress, panic, anxiety, or disorder triggers the extreme adrenaline, special medication will alleviate the signs. Beta-blockers that will bind to the heart's receptors will prevent the occurrence of heart failure caused by too much secretion of the stress hormones.

Conclusion

Adrenaline rushes occur when you are confronted with an abrupt threat. The potential danger can perhaps range from a barking dog, family or job stress, or from a person trying to fight against you. As a result, the blood pressure and heart rate become elevated which is not good when not properly controlled. Manage your own adrenaline by rightly handling your moments of stress and your response to nerve- racking circumstances. Control your thoughts and your words to put limitations to your emerging adrenaline.

Chapter 9- How Does Adrenaline Affect your Body?

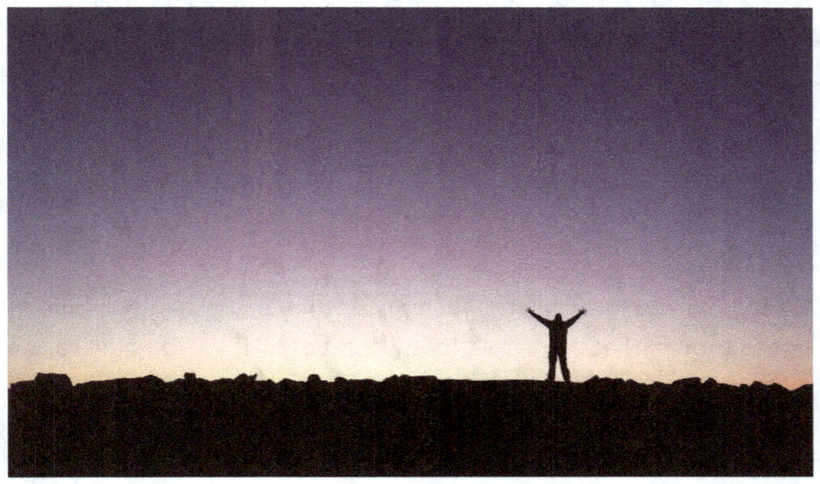

To lose weight, one must understand how the body works. In order for a person to lose weight, they need to have a certain healthy diet and do a lot of physical activity.

A very popular way of shedding pounds is by doing high or low intensity cardio. But did you know that you can lose weight fast if you have a better understanding of Adrenaline?

How adrenaline is related to fat loss, you may ask. Adrenaline is actually a hormone that regulates your heart rate. It helps in the process in the fat breakdown. How? I'll explain by giving an example.

A study was done with two groups of women, all obese. One group was asked to a 20 minute interval training using a bike. They were asked to do 8 second high intensity cycling followed by 12 seconds recovery.

The second group was asked to perform 40 minutes of slow and light intensity cardio. Both groups were asked to do this three times a week for fifteen weeks. The results were stunning. The group who did a 20 minute training showed impressive weight loss results. And the second group who did cardio double the time that the first had no weight loss.

Doing interval training helps you release adrenaline, and as already mentioned above; adrenaline breaks down fat stores and burns them.

It can help you lose weight much faster than doing steady cardio. It doesn't mean that you won't lose weight at all if you do only cardio exercises, you will. It just won't be as fast and evident as doing interval training.

Here is another fact about adrenaline, once it gets you going and released in your body, it can be in your blood for hours. That being said, you are burning fat really fast that no amount of intense cardio or heavy weight lifting can do.

Another way that adrenaline helps you lose weight is that it actually decreases your appetite. That means if on a regular day of workout wherein you will want to eat more after the tiring activity, adrenaline does the opposite.

Knowing all these facts can help you choose the right kind of workout. But whenever you are trying to lose weight, it is still important to consider the kind of diet you have.

More than anything, being healthy inside and out is more important that looking good in a bikini. So load up on those yummy veggies, skip that highly tempting cheeseburger and fries meal and drink at least 8 glasses of water each day for a better looking, healthier you!

Aside from adrenaline, there are other hormones that are used slimming. Some of the most popular of these hormones are the thyroid hormone and the appetite suppressing hormones Leptin and Ghrelin.

Thyroid Hormones for Losing Weight

Thyroid hormones have potential benefits for weight loss because it has the ability to increase the metabolism. This happens when the thyroid gland produces an excessive amount of the thyroid hormone. This state is referred to as hypothyroidism which can also mean under-production of the hormone. It is has been that while your under the state hypothyroidism, you can lose as much as 10 to 15 pounds.

The Application of thyroid hormones for dropping excess weight has been extensively studied and results provided strong indications that the hormone is effective. In fact, it was found out that the more severe the hyperthyroidism, the more it is effective for reducing weight.

Thyroid Hormones Safety Issues

Thyroid hormones may have been found helpful for weight loss but it has dangers that should be considered. One of these is the moment the excessive thyroid hormone production ceases, the lost weight is likely to be gained back. Another safety issue is the possible protein loss that accompanies fat loss.

Also, hyperthyroidism increases the need for increased calorie intake and it is possible that dieters will it difficult to reduce calorie consumption when they stop using the hormone.

It is recommended that the use of the Thyroid hormone for weight loss should be under the supervision of a doctor. First of all a doctor can give valuable advice on whether the dieter is healthy enough to engage in exercises, or diet or supplements are appropriate.

Leptin and Ghrelin Hormones

Leptin and ghrelin are appetite controlling hormones that send signals to the brain which decides whether the fats and calories consumed are stored as triglycerides or used as energy.

Weight loss benefits

The effect of the two hormones on weight loss has been studied and it was the amount of leptin and ghrelin before a weight loss diet is started can determine a dieter's capability for sustaining weight loss. It seems that when there are more leptin and less ghrelin in the body, weight loss is difficult to sustain.

How to Make the Hormones Work

There are a lot of things still unknown about these hormones although researchers agree that they are powerful fat metabolizers and appetite hormones. Scientists, however, know that a pill containing these hormones has no apparent effect on weight loss and that the only way it could be of benefit for weight loss is to change dietary habits and lifestyles.

Four dietary changes are recommended: no eating after 7 PM, five small meals a day, protein loaded breakfast, and no refined carbs or sugar.

It will be difficult for dieters to implement the changes without encountering problems. However, the human body works at peak levels on low sugar and carb eaten over a period of time and while some modifications are allowed, permanent weight reduction targets can be met only by controlling leptin and ghrelin, the two appetite hormones.

Adrenaline rush, it's a term you must have heard of plenty of times. Adrenaline is a hormone that the body produces during stressful, exciting or physically demanding situations.

The hormone constricts the blood vessels, expands air passages and increases the heart rate. The adrenaline rush that results from this provide your body with an energy boost that allows you to immediately respond to the situation or situations you are faced with.

How Fitness Benefits From Adrenaline

Adrenaline has decisive effect on your fitness because with the additional energy that it supplies, you will be able to perform the most physically demanding routines. Thus, in many weight loss and fitness diet programs, adrenaline boosting foods will not be left out. They will have the foods with the nutrients – lean protein and complex carbohydrates – that boost adrenaline levels in the body.

Other Benefits

Recently there has been an increased interest in the use of adrenaline not only for weight loss and fitness. Sometimes people simply feel weary with all the activities they have to attend to. Adrenaline that is contained in many energy boosting products re-invigorates their tiring systems.

Aside from the energy and the benefits it provides to dieters and fitness adherents, adrenaline is also used for medical purposes. It is known to reduce symptoms of serious allergic reactions and alleviates the sufferings of people undergoing anaphylactic shocks.

Dangers of Adrenaline Excess

However, an excessive amount of adrenaline in your body is to be avoided as it can result to some serious health problems. You will be fidgety and tense, and sleep will not come easy. In children, it can cause abnormal behaviors. This is the reason why drinking too much coffee or taking drugs is not safe. The disproportionate amounts of adrenaline produced by these activities will keep your body extra alert and tense and when your body is kept in this condition for long periods, it can be damaged.

There are several ways of reducing the amount of adrenaline circulating in your body that affects the smooth functioning of your systems. Some drugs can do that, but the best way is to engage in exercises like walking and other types of exercises. Exercise eases your tense muscles, relieves your insomnia and calms your agitated nervous system.

Exercises to work off excess adrenaline

One of the more popular exercises that people engage in to specifically lessen adrenaline is the boot camp. This type of routine involves the use of car tires, ropes, balls and cones. Done in groups, it is fun and relaxing. Of course, it is also a wonderful way of burning calories and getting fit.

It is obvious that fitness programs have significant impact on your adrenaline levels. First, it is easier to observe fitness exercises when you have adequate energy and adrenaline provides you that. So in fitness as well as weight loss diets adrenaline boosting foods are always primary considerations. Second, issues with over-production of adrenaline that causes you some problems are easily solved by simple exercises.

Chapter 10 - The Role of Nutrition for your Fitness

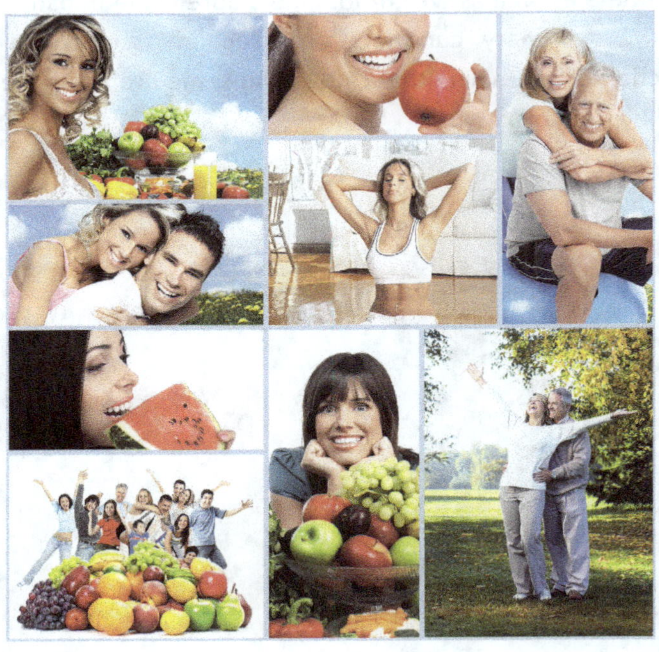

With people focused on weight loss and slimming, health is often left out from many weight loss strategies. Slimming has become the primary concern, which when you look at it more closely, is unfortunate.

From whatever angle you look at the slimming issue, you will always come to the conclusion that there is no such thing as slimming without health.

Of course, some of the slimming programs that promise you quick results like drastically reduced diets can give you the figure you desire, but you have no guarantee the weight problem will not recur and the cost sometimes is a bit too high.

The Best Way to Slim Down

You have to admit that prioritizing nutrition or a nutritionally balanced diet and fitness is the best way of sliming. Your body has inherent mechanisms for preventing abnormalities like excessive weight and all you have to do is to make sure these mechanisms are working properly.

Different nutrients do different valuable things for your body systems. Calories are for energy, fiber helps the liver and metabolism to work well, vitamins and minerals generally are for maintenance and operations. It is when you do not take enough or a bit too much of a certain nutrient that your body stops working as efficiently as it should.

For example, when you take in more calories than you need, your body converts the excess calories into fat tissues and from there a whole of range of negative things can happen not only to your health but to your physical appearance as well.

Proper nutrition allows the body to work properly so that health problems like excess poundage are prevented. If nutrition is preventive it can also be curative because once you get your body systems working properly again it can, with some assistance, remove your unwanted weight.

Fitness Workout: How It Induces Slimming

The assistance that you need to provide comes in the form of fitness exercises and, of course, a diet that is calorie reduced and contains all the other helpful nutrients that will make your systems work more efficiently.

Compared to slimming pills or crash diets that make you undergo deprivations that most often harm your body, solving a slimming problem using a nutritionally balanced diet is admittedly slow but when your over-all health is at stake the speed with which you slim down should take a back seat.

Fitness exercise also plays a crucial role in slimming. It is probably the lean body and the abs you are after, but it does a lot for getting your weight back into normal and making you slim. Workouts require energy and your diet providing fewer calories, there is only one source of energy where you can get it – from the fat deposits in your body.

Lean muscles that only fitness exercises can develop requires less energy to maintain compared to fats. Thus, you experience reduced cravings for food, especially for calorie rich foods. Fitness exercises are actually one of the better of staying slim or getting slim.

Slimming has spawned numerous programs – fad diets, hormonal treatments, natural methods, yoga, and surgical methods. There is always something new in each of these.

Every so often, some new kind of diet that is supposed to remove excess weight fast and is easy is introduced in the market and people with weight issues would try it. There is never a diet regime too difficult to do as long as it promises a speedy and definite solution.

Going Organic

Lately slimming diets are increasingly becoming non-pharmaceutical. This shift from pharmaceutical products is the result of the growing awareness of people that slimming dangers are likely to be prevented with the use of organic solutions or concoctions.

Organic foods that are proven to possess energy boosting, metabolism changing and calorie blocking or carb absorption properties seems to be the areas of interest in slimming these days.

Most of these of products are supplements, of course, but they interest a lot people because they can lose extra pounds without resorting to diet plans that force them to endure intense hunger pangs and food cravings.

Often weight loss supplements are extracts from fruits and herbs. There is no lack of such products in the market and their number continue to increase as more and more fruits and herbal are discovered to contain slimming properties.

Surgical Procedures

For those who have money to spare and who have exhausted all other means the area of slimming interests are the fast acting programs basically surgical procedures.

These days, wide incisions are no longer necessary as most surgeries are done via laparoscopic procedures where all that's required is a tiny incision for inserting of camera and tools for melting the accumulated fat layers. It is estimated that around 200,000 people undergo weight loss surgeries each year.

The latest method slimming surgery is the Gastric Plication, which does not actually remove the fats but drastically reduces the appetite by placing folds in the stomach. It is a method that is minimally invasive.

Weight Loss Massage

There are two types of weight loss massage. One performed by a machine, another by a human. The first is accomplished by applying a machine that gives the body a massage while applying heat. There are many kinds of massage for weight loss performed by humans, most supplemented by herbal lotions.

Hormone Injections

The human body has many hormones which are capable of speeding– up fat burning, improving the metabolic process, boosting energy levels, and other things that help reduce weight Many companies producing weight loss products are constantly studying these hormones and coming up with products based on them.

Fat Clubs

Then there are Fat clubs which are meant to provide adequate support to dieters. They are with people with the same problem so they can relate and sympathize. Of course, they have to follow specific slimming programs and guidelines.

The point of these clubs is dieters are more motivated to succeed because they are doing the same things and the success of one motivates the other to strive even harder.

CHAPTER 11- MUST HAVE FITTER BODY – 10 REASONS

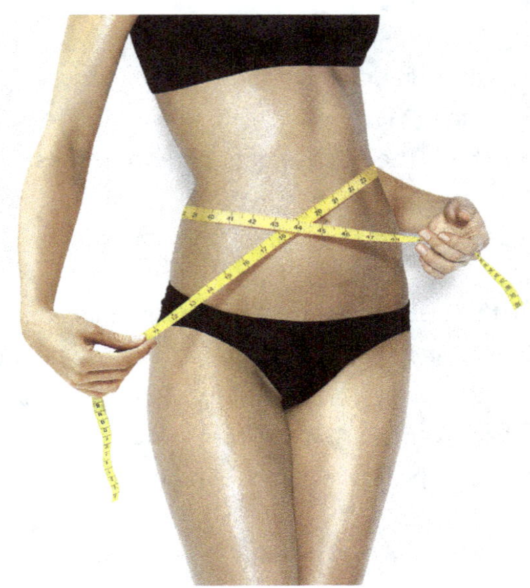

There are several reasons why you need to lose weight. Aside from getting a sexier and healthier body, you also get to enjoy so many things. You may not see it by now, but time will come that you will appreciate your decision to lose weight.

However, working out and eating the right foods are easier said than done. Your lack of time and motivation may drive you away from doing all these things. So, to help you keep going, here are the top reasons why you need to stay healthy and fit.

Reason #1: Longer Life

Who does not want to live longer? Sure, you would love to see your kids grow and have their own families, play with your grandchildren and of course, enjoy your retirement benefits. With this, you need to have a fitter body for you to live longer. Just focus on a balance diet and healthy lifestyle. Avoid bad habits like smoking, drinking alcohol and eating processed foods.

Reason #2: More energy

Doing exercise can sustain your momentum and keep you going all throughout the day. More so, it can make you feel better since regular exercise fuels the release of good endorphins.

Reason #3: Lesser Risk of Acquiring Diseases

This is one of the good reasons why you should maintain a fitter body. Healthy diet and regular exercise can stimulate the release of toxins and reduce free radicals. Moreover, a healthy lifestyle reduce the risk of acquiring diseases including heart disease, diabetes, high blood pressure, cancer and other health issues.

Reason #4: Less medical expenses

Keeping your body healthy allows you to save money by not visiting your doctor regularly and buying medicines.

Reason #5: Better Self-confidence

Obesity can affect your confidence. Hence, it is important to keep your body fit to maintain and improve your self-esteem. You surely don't want to feel insecure all your life, right?

Reason #6: Improved Overall Look and Aura

You look a lot better when you are fit and healthy. The appearance of your skin will improve and you will have that overall glow. Additionally, you can wear anything you want making you more stylish and chic.

Reason #7: Better Mental Health

When you do regular exercise, your mental health improves. You experience less stress and depression. You feel more relax and problem-free.

Reason # 8: Being More Sociable

When you feel good about yourself, you become more confident and willing to socialize. You gain new friends and enjoy life even more with your loved ones.

Reason #9: Improved Sex Life

Healthy diet and lifestyle allows you to enjoy and have a better sex life. Furthermore, regular exercise can help reduce the risk of erectile deficiency.

Reason # 10: Thrive Instead Of Just Surviving

If you still want to enjoy life when you turn 80 or 90, you need to keep your body fit. Don't let yourself be one of those bedridden oldies. Isn't it great if you still can blow out your candles then hit the dance floor afterwards?

These are the 10 really good reasons why you should go for a fitter body. Hopefully, they are convincing enough for you to hit the gym everyday and eat a balanced diet. Besides, it is still you who will benefit at the end. Stay fit!

CHAPTER 12- THE TRUE ESSENCE OF A FITTER BODY

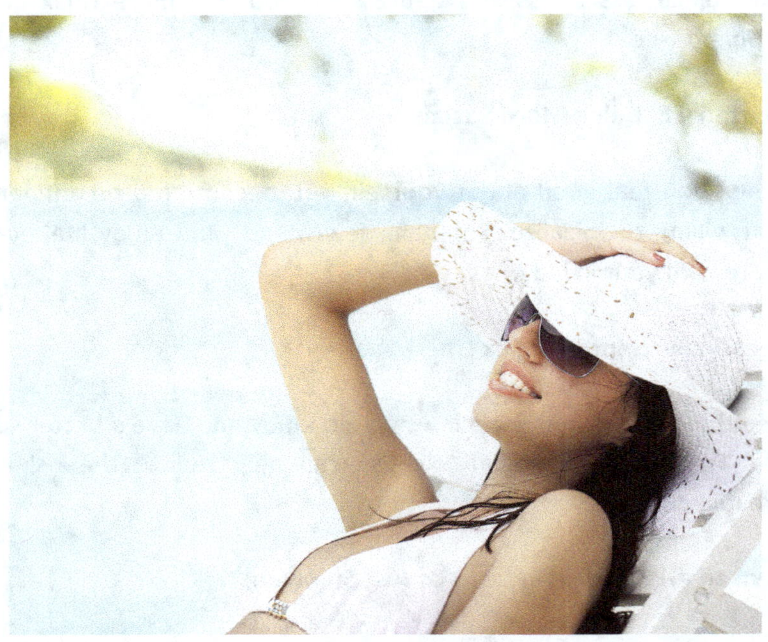

Good health doesn't just mean looking great. There's more to it than that. A person can have a really toned body but can still not be considered healthy. So stop looking at the mirror and actually pay close attention to what your mind and body are telling you.

Being healthy means having a good state of the mind, body and spirit. There are five aspects of health. These are physical, mental, emotional, spiritual and social. You will learn more about all of these as you read on.

Starting With the Physical Health

Being physically healthy means a person's body is strong enough to combat different diseases. Having a physically healthy body is not a piece of cake and to get there, a person would need to work on it.

This means regularly exercising or staying active and eating nutritious food. A good sign that of being physically healthy is when a person doesn't easily get sick and is always full of energy.

Mental Health

Mental Health is a person's ability to use their brain each day. Which means being alert and can handle situations where thinking is involved without easily getting stressed. It's being able to concentrate on task at hand and while doing so, make smart decisions, being creative and digesting knowledge and understanding of things around.

Emotional Health

Emotional Health is when a person feels good about herself, the people around her, and everything that involves her life. When one is emotionally healthy, this means they are in control of their feelings and don't easily break down when something terrible happens such as being rejected, defeated or neglected. They can also handle happiness and success in stride. Incidentally, if a person is emotionally healthy, they are less likely to experience minor sickness that one gets when stressed such as migraines or ulcer.

Spiritual Health

Spiritual Health is something that is harder to explain and even understand. Not to be confused with any religious belief, spiritual health is how a person expresses his or her values. It's how they exercise the spirit. Knowing what's right and what's wrong and applying it in their everyday life. Being kind to people, living creatures on earth and the environment is what defines a spiritually healthy being.

Social Health is how a person is maintaining a good relationship (if not good, then respectful) with others. If you are considerate of the feelings of other people in your life then you are a socially healthy

person. Are you a good son or daughter? A good husband or wife? A good student? A good neighbor? A good friend? A good citizen? Do you do your duties and contribute into making their life better? Do you influence people for the best?

If you have enemies, do you hold grudges or are open to forgiveness? These are some of the factors that determine whether you are socially healthy or not.

In conclusion, health is more than just being free from diseases. You need to balance all five aspects in order to feel peace and long term happiness.

ABOUT THE AUTHOR

Alice Campbell is very good in her field as a fitness instructor. She conducted several fitness classes that have a wide range of different programs to cater different needs of her students. Alice believes that everyone can achieve their desired body. That is why she laid out various meals plans, workout schedule, authored books and even created instructional videos to help and inspire others.

Alice, together with her 3 kids, live in Oklahoma.